Simplifying Weight Loss

Weight Loss Simplified And Made Real For Laymen

A. Gumise

Introduction

Are you tired of stepping on the scale and seeing the same numbers?

Do you feel like nothing is working, no matter how hard you try and are looking for a weight loss formula that works without making you lose your mind in the process?

If you have answered YES, this book is for you!

Trying to lose weight can feel so exhausting when you don't see any progress. However, it doesn't have to be that way. You can turn things around, enjoy the process of weight loss, and effectively see those pounds coming off by directing your efforts to certain things.

And this book seeks to help you to understand what those things are so you can effectively propel yourself to effortless weight loss!

The book will help you understand what is going on in your body and give you practical methods to cut those pounds and keep them off once and for all!

What's more, the book will give you the much-needed motivation and morale that will hold you by the hand until you achieve your desired weight and stick to a healthy fit lifestyle.

Let's begin!

Table of Contents

Chapter 1: How And Why We Gain Weight

It is easy to blindly follow diets, exercise routines, juice fasts, and so on to lose weight without even understanding how your body is gaining weight in the first place. There are so many factors as to why we might be gaining weight, and unless you deal with it from the core, your efforts will be pretty much that, just efforts.

So how do our bodies put on those extra pounds?

How The Body Puts On Weight

We are what we eat.

For the body to put on weight, there must be that aspect of eating, regardless of why you are putting on weight, be it hormones or being sedentary.

Picture this...

You've just had a burger. As you chew on the well-cooked patty and crunchy lettuce, digestion has already started in your mouth through the saliva, which breaks down starch into sugar. This sugar, together with the rest of the ingredients, move down into your belly. Here hydrochloric acid and pepsin (an enzyme responsible for protein digestion) break down the food further to form a substance known as chyme. This mixture moves to your duodenum, and the bile dissolves the fat, which thins out the chyme, making it easier to absorb. Again, the enzymes in the pancreas enter the duodenum to further break down the proteins, fat, and sugar.

So now that your burger has been completely dissolved into liquid form, it is time for the patty (protein), fat (oil/grease), and sugar (from all ingredients containing it) to say bye-bye to each other.

1. *So, where does the sugar go?*

The sugar pumps directly into your bloodstream, and different organs absorb the sugar they need and pass it by. Excess of it is stored in the muscle and liver as glycogen to be used for energy whenever your blood sugar levels are low, while some go to the brain.

2. *And where does the fat go?*

The fat moves to the bloodstream first and then goes to the liver. The liver burns some of it, and some is converted into substances such as cholesterol. The excess is sent into the fat cells, where it waits until it is needed.

3. And what about the patty?

The patty, i.e., the protein, is broken down into building blocks popularly known as peptides. This is further broken down into amino acids, which are absorbed through the lining of the small intestine and then into the bloodstream. Some of these amino acids add up to the protein stores while some, **get this,** are converted into sugars and fats, which then follow the paths described.

So what do all of these digestions have in common? As you can see, any food you consume in whichever form, when consumed excessively, is stored in the body (fat cells) waiting to be utilized.

So why do we have excess food in the first place:

Where All The Extra Calories That Lead To Weight Gain Come From

Storage of excess fats can happen for several reasons:

Overeating

This is a no brainer. If you overeat, you have more food available for conversion into fats, which are stored in the body - regardless of the macronutrient consumed. For instance, many people believe that they can consume as much protein as they want to because it is instantaneously converted into muscle, but as you have already seen, this is far from the truth.

As long as you eat more calories than you use during the day, then you will gain weight.

Eating unhealthily

Even if all the food you consume ends up as fat, what you consume is also as important. Junk food contains high amounts of fat and or sugar even in the smallest portions. A typical slice of pizza contains around 250 to 300 calories! Compare this with 100 calories of a plate of veggies (say a salad comprising of cucumber, lettuce, and carrots). Plus, a plate of veggies is way more filling compared to junk food because of the fiber content. With junk, you will keep eating and eating and will finally feel full after consuming crazy amounts of calories.

Remaining sedentary

So you wake up in the morning, take a shower, get coffee and a donut from Starbucks, then get a bus/Uber to work. You sit at your desk for about 4 hours where the most motion you made was waving at your colleagues while they were coming in. During lunch break, you get yourself a hotdog and maybe a milkshake to go because you are in a hurry to get back to your desk. You get there and sit for more hours as you continue working. After work, you Uber home, and since you feel drained, you decide to order take out (because who has the time to defrost the chicken). Your take out arrives, and you feast as you watch something on Netflix until you doze off.

Now imagine this kind of life on a loop. If you just sit around, whether it's at home or at the office, without doing anything much, then you are bound to put on some pounds., your body needs to be in some sort of motion to burn calories

Medication

This is one factor that you can't do much about because you can't stop taking important medication simply because you are gaining some pounds. Certain drugs in your medicine cabinet may be the culprits to your weight gain, such as insulin, steroids, antipsychotic drugs, among others.

What you can do here is to ensure that you are following a healthy and balanced diet and staying as active as possible.

It Is All About Calories!

The body uses energy (obtained from the food or drinks you take) to perform everything, from the invisible processes within the cells to the visible ones like breathing, walking, talking, thinking, running, lifting stuff, and much more.

Just like any machine, how much energy it uses at a given time will depend on how many processes/activities it is engaging in and the energy requirements for the activities in question. If what the body is doing needs more energy, you burn a lot of calories. And if what you are doing does not really expend a lot of energy, you burn fewer calories.

This essentially means if you over-fuel your body by eating foods that generate a lot of energy (more than what the body needs), there will be more energy than it can use to perform the different activities. This extra fuel has to go somewhere.

The body, in its wisdom, through evolution, has developed mechanisms for that! It converts the excess fuel into a form that can be stored in the body for use when the supply of fuel is low. There are 2 forms of storage; glycogen and fatty acids and glycerol. If glucose and proteins are in excess, they may be converted to glycerol in the liver then stored in the liver and muscle cells. Glycogen stores have a limited capacity, though. So if there is still extra glucose, protein, or fat, they are converted to fatty acids, and glycerol is then transported to different fat stores around the body.

This is how we gain weight – from the excesses of the calories we get from different foods and drinks.

Let me refer you to an equation that you will help you understand everything:

1. If the calories you've taken in are equal to the calories you've used up, **you maintain weight**

2. If the calories you've taken in are more than the calories you've used up, **you gain weight.**

3. And if the calories you've taken in are less than the calories you've used up, **you lose weight**

Your goal in your journey to weight loss should be to make the most of the third formula or at least maintain your current weight in whichever means possible. If you make the most of the third formula, you create what is referred to as calorie deficit, a situation where the energy from the food you've eaten is lower than how much your body actually needs, something that pushes it to start using the stored energy that we talked about earlier.

With that in mind, how many calories should you be eating generally in a day to prevent this excessive storage of fat?

Your Caloric Needs

As we have already established, you need to burn calories for fat loss to happen (or consume fewer calories to create a caloric deficit).

Generally, you need around 1500 to 2000 calories to maintain your bodyweight if you are a woman and 2000 to 2500 for men.

You will need to consume about **<u>1200 calories (women) or 1800 calories for men per day</u>** to lose weight.

As this is a general figure, you can use the following method to get how many calories you need in a day to lose weight:

#1. Calculate your BMR

Your basal metabolic rate gives you the number of calories your body needs to function if you are inactive or less active. You can use this equation known as the Mifflin-St Jeor equation to find BMR:

$$10(m) + 6.25(h) - 5(a) + s$$

m- Weight in kilograms

h- Height in cm

a- Age

s- Sex (for male, add 5 and for female, less 161)

4. Tips regarding the formula

If you have your weight in pounds, multiply it by 2.2 to get it in kg

If you have your height in inches, divide it by 2.54 to get it in cm.

#2. Factor in your activity level

Unless you are on bed rest, it is not possible to go all day without even lifting a finger or moving a bit in the house. After calculating your BMR, you can now use the Harris-Benedict Formula to determine your caloric needs in relation to your activity level. The formula narrates that you multiply your BMR with your suitable activity factor where:

5. Sedentary- Little to no exercise multiply BMR by 1.2

6. Lightly active- Light exercise/ sports for 1 to 3 days in a week, multiply BMR by 1.375

7. Moderately active- If you engage in moderate exercise/sports for like 3 to 5 days a week, multiply BMR by 1.55

8. Very active - Hard exercise or sports for 6 days a week, multiply BMR by 1.725

9. Extra active- If you engage in very hard exercise/sport or have a hard physical job such as construction, multiply BMR by 1.9

Whatever you get is the number of calories you need each day.

Pro tip: If you are not good with numbers, you can use these calculators – all you need to do is to input the figures - the websites will generate the results for you!

https://www.calculator.net/calorie-calculator.html

https://www.mayoclinic.org/healthy-lifestyle/weight-loss/in-depth/calorie-calculator/itt-20402304

https://www.acefitness.org/education-and-resources/lifestyle/tools-calculators/daily-caloric-needs-estimate-calculator/

Chapter 2: You Are What You Eat

It doesn't matter how much you exercise; if your diet is trash, you won't see much progress - this is why cleaning up your diet comes first.

What To Eat (And What Not To!)

If you want to lose weight and keep it off for good, then there are some foods you will have to do away with, for good (or have them in small amounts, infrequently).

Your general rule should be '**<u>Eat clean, healthy, and real food and avoid processed and refined products.</u>**'

Before you pick out a meal/cook a meal, ask yourself what the ingredients are. Does the meal contain more processed ingredients than real ingredients? If so, try and substitute the processed ingredients with real ones, e.g., you can switch out pasta for zucchini noodles.

Generally, avoid these foods:

Pastries, cakes, and cookies- These often contain crazy amounts of added sugar, refined flour, and trans fat (but not always). These foods are also high in calories but are not filling, so you are bound to feel hungry soon after consuming them - this increases your caloric intake.

Most Fruit Juices - Fun fact: the fruit juices you see at the supermarket have very little to do with the fruit displayed nicely on the bottles. Some are usually just filled with flavoring and added sugars, and while there are really fruit juices from the real fruits, these aren't that healthy either. Fruit juices contain as many calories and sugar, as soda or even more while having zero fiber content, meaning you consume larger quantities easily. Therefore, just stick to whole fruits.

Candy bars - A candy bar is a non-nutritious small package filled with added sugar, oils, and refined flour. A small candy bar can contain up to 300 calories! I know. Just avoid these

Potato chips and French fries - Their main ingredient, whole potatoes, are very healthy and filling but potato chips and french fries aren't. Both are high in calories, and overeating them is so easy - ever thrown your hand in your chip bag to grab some chips only to find nothing? That's what I'm talking about.

Pizza - It is so easy to just order a pizza and have it delivered within minutes, but this isn't a good thing. Commercially made pizzas are so unhealthy with their crazy amounts of cheese, processed meat, and refined flour. Try homemade pizzas and pizza sauce instead, or find a place that makes healthier options.

Ice cream - Yes I know. As delicious as this treat is, it is not as healthy. Most types are loaded with sugars and are high in calories. A small portion every now and then is okay, but we both know that self-control is hard to muster when it comes to ice cream. You can always try making your own ice cream with less sugar and healthier options such as fruit and full-fat yogurt.

Alcohol (especially beer)

Have you ever heard of a "beer belly"? Some pints of lager contains about 180 calories while providing no nutrition except a buzz and abdominal fat. Drinking alcohol in moderation seems to be fine, or you could go for other types of alcohol such as wine.

With that in mind, opt to eat foods such as:

Meats - Chicken, beef, lamb, etc.

Veggies - Kale, spinach, cabbage, etc.

Tubers - Sweet potatoes, arrow roots, etc.

Whole fruits - Apples, mangoes, pears, kiwi, etc.

Whole grains - Millet, oatmeal, barley, brown rice, etc.

Spices and herbs - Turmeric, parsley, coriander, pepper, etc.

Seeds and nuts - Cashews, sunflower seeds, almonds, etc.

Legumes - Beans, peanuts, etc.

Dairy - Cheese, yogurt, milk, etc.

Basically, eat anything that is real and has nutritional value - your diet isn't limited to the foods mentioned above.

Portion control is key

Even with your change in diet, you must exercise portion control to actually lose weight. Eating a whole chicken simply because it is healthy will prove to be counterproductive. Portion control ensures that you create a calorie deficit, which means that your body has to burn stored up fat for energy, leading to weight loss. The point here is to give your body exactly what it needs - no more no less.

Tips for portion control

Meal prep- Meal prepping is one great way to ensure that you stick to a healthy menu. What makes us eat out or order take out is usually the lack of ready food in the house so imagine if you always have something in the fridge waiting for you to devour it. Take a day or two to prepare various healthy and balanced meals and store them in the fridge.

It's always a good idea to fill up on veggies- Veggies help you exercise portion control without so much effort as they contain fewer calories and are so filling. As you serve your food, have more veggies than other types of food.

Read nutritional labels - Read all the labels to understand what your food constitutes and the recommended serving size. If you already understand your caloric needs (which I assume you do by now), you will be able to figure out the amount of food you should be eating. Also, check the labels for the amount of sugars, proteins, carbs, etc. contained in that food and determine if it is good for your overall goals.

Take it slow- If you are used to eating fast, it can be a bit hard to retrain yourself but keep in mind that the slower you eat, the more likely you are to notice that you are full before finishing. You can try and chew your food more, or have sips of water between bites, or set your utensils down after a bite for a specific amount of time; any trick that will work for you.

Serve in smaller plates - We usually feel like we are supposed to finish all the food on our plates, so using smaller plates gives you that satisfaction while keeping your portions in check. This is way better than eating on a larger plate and leaving some food behind, which usually makes you feel like you haven't enjoyed a full meal.

Get yourself some small bowls and plates - and serving spoons too!

Water up- Drinking water before a meal helps you eat less and lose weight faster. When you are dehydrated, you feel the urge to eat more because you are both hungry and thirsty. Actually, sometimes when we are thirsty, we tend to think that we are hungry. Therefore, the next time you are hungry, gobble down a glass of water and wait 30 minutes. If you are still hungry, then have your meal/snack.

Different diets to try

In addition to eating right, there are many great diets out there that you can try out. The secret is finding what works for you and sticking to it.

These diets and eating methods include:

The Keto Diet

Also known as LCHF (low carb high fat), this diet entails the consumption of high amounts of fats, moderate proteins, and low amounts of carbs with the goal being to get the body into a state of what's referred to as nutritional ketosis.

With this diet, your body stops relying on glucose as its main source of energy. It starts relying on ketones (obtained from the breakdown of fat) as the main energy source. When the fats you have consumed are depleted, your body then starts burning body fat for energy. This essentially means your body is burning fat 24/7 (how awesome is this!)

General Guidelines

For this diet, 75% of your calorie intake should come from fats, 20% should come from protein, and not more than 5% should come from carbs (you should have just about 20 to 50 grams of carbs a day).

Just as you are watching your carb intake, you should also watch your protein intake (remember protein also gets converted into glucose). Your protein intake should be around 0.7-0.9 grams per pound of body weight. So if you are 162 pounds, your protein intake will be around 129 grams a day. The rest of your caloric needs should be met by fat.

Alkaline Diet

This diet is based on the concept that eating alkaline forming foods (those that leave behind an alkaline ash in the body, with a pH of 7 and above) helps maintain a balanced pH in the body and that acid forming foods (those whose residue in the body has a pH of below 7) throws pH out of balance, leading to poor health.

General Guidelines

This diet encourages consumption of healthy food options such as veggies, fruits, seeds, legumes, etc. which are alkaline-forming and discourages foods such as aerated beverages and processed foods - this can aid in weight loss.

In detail, you should focus on eating whole foods and drinking alkalizing beverages such as green tea, spring water, and ginger root or water with a splash of lemon or lime.

Meat, fish, essential fats, pasta, and other grains should be consumed in small amounts, whereas white sugar, artificial foods, caffeine, and white flour should be eliminated completely. And always use high-quality oil and fats such as olive oil, coconut oil, and avocado oil.

Paleo Diet

This diet takes you back to eating the way our ancestors used to, you know, real whole food. The diet aims to go back to eating in a way that is meant for humans, as its belief is that our bodies have been mismatched genetically to the modern diet through farming. Farming established foods such as grains, dairy, legumes, and processed foods, which are believed to be the main cause of diabetes, obesity, and heart disease today.

General Guidelines

Your general rule here should be, 'If a caveman didn't eat it, neither should I'.

Ideally, you should eat foods such as meats, nuts, seeds, fruits, fish, spices and herbs, oils, eggs, and fresh vegetables. You can also drink herbal teas, kombucha, coconut water, and fresh juice from veggies and fruits consumed with the pulp.

Avoid foods such as grains, legumes, dairy, refined oils and refined flours and sugar, soda and sweetened beverages, artificial sweeteners, and salt.

Intermittent Fasting

This is a pattern of eating where you cycle between periods of fasting and periods of eating with the aim being that you get your body into what's referred to as the fasted state.

With intermittent fasting, your body alternates between a fed state and a fasted state. The point of this is that when in a fasted state, your body can utilize body fat more effectively as it gets a break from other processes of digestion such as the breakdown of glucose, etc. This body fat is otherwise inaccessible when you are always in the fed state.

General Guidelines

There are different methods to do intermittent fasting, with the popular ones being:

- Eat stop eat - This method involves fasting for 24 hours straight for 1 or 2 days a week and then eating normally for the rest of the days. This method aims to reduce your overall caloric intake in a week and push your body into the fasted state, which promotes consistent fat burning.

- 16/8 - This is where you fast for 16 hours a day and squeeze all your meals within the remaining 8 hours. With this method, most people prefer skipping breakfast as part of their fast, which makes it easier to follow. You have to fast daily while following the 16/8 method.

- Warrior diet - With this method, you fast for 20 hours a day and have a feeding window of 4 hours. This feeding window should be in the evening, just like the warriors who used to hunt all day and feast in the evenings. The fast is also carried out every day.

- Alternate day fasting - For this method, you get to eat every other day - you fast for 36 hours, have a 12 hour feeding period, and then fast again. You can choose to have no food or have around 500 calories during the fasting window.

Don't stop at following diets though. As already mentioned, one of the ways to increase your body's calorie requirements is exercising. Let's learn more about exercising.

Chapter 3: Move Your Body!

When you combine your great eating habits with exercise, weight loss becomes effortless. There are so many ways to get your body in motion - don't just think about contemporary jogging at 5.am in the morning, although that's one way to do it.

So how can you exercise to burn that fat?

The Basics Of Exercising

Regardless of the exercise that you are doing, follow the following general guidelines:

Frequency of workouts

If you really want to see results, you will need to exercise at least 4 to 5 times a week. But don't worry, you can work up to this.

Begin by working out for 2 days a week and slowly increase the days as you progress. You can choose any days of the week but if you are working out 2 times a week, try and not make those days consecutive - for instance, you can work out on a Monday and a Saturday.

Duration of workouts

Sorry, but there isn't one duration that is ideal for everybody. This is because a work out can comprise of warm-ups, cool downs, stretching, cardio, weight training, and so much more. But generally, your workout shouldn't be less than 30 minutes. If you engage in HIIT (High-Intensity Interval Training), the duration may be shorter (even 7 minutes of HIIT is considered enough for a session).

Eating for a workout

You should not work out right after a meal - you might even feel sick doing this. Wait for at least 2 hours if you just had a meal and wait for 15-20 minutes to eat after a workout to give your body time to recover.

Change your routine

If you've ever worked out and all of a sudden, you got to wondering why the exercises are so easy, then you probably weren't changing routine. Our bodies are made in a way that, over time, they get used to any form of exertion, so doing the same exercises may not give the same results over time.

Aim to change your exercises every 4 weeks.

The Workout Options

1: Cardio

Cardio is any form of exercise that gets you sweating and gets your heart rate up. In reality, any form of exercise can be considered as cardio, although there are many different variations.

You can do the following cardio exercises:

Jogging

Running at a steady, moderate pace is a sure way to burn some calories and fat. You can choose to run outside or run on a treadmill. Just make sure to wear appropriate shoes so that you don't hurt yourself.

Aim to run for 30 to 60 minutes a week (this translates to 5 to 10 minutes a day).

Climbing stairs

Climbing stairs is another great way to burn fat and burn muscle (the higher you have to lift your leg, the more muscle you build). Again, you can utilize the stair climber at your gym or climb up and down a flight of stairs - both work great. You can do this exercise for about 5 minutes combined with other exercises (30 seconds then active rest of 30 seconds).

Jumping rope

Jumping rope is an all-round cardio. Not only does it get your heart rate up to burn calories (up to 500 calories in 30 minutes!), it also enhances your footwork, coordination, and shoulder strength.

Since it's a bit hard to jump rope for 30 minutes straight, you can try and do slow and fast jumps at intervals or jump for a minute, rest for 30 seconds and repeat until you are done.

Cycling

Riding your bike is a fun way to get your cardio on. Other variations of cycling include using a stationary bike or enrolling in a spin class. Indoor cycling or spin class (vigorous) will have you burning close to 1000 calories an hour, while moderate cycling will burn you around half of that.

Try and alternate intensities to build your endurance. You can go really intense for a couple of minutes and then slow down for a minute and then continue for as long as you can. If you are riding a bike outside, challenge yourself by riding in rough terrain or up a hill for more intensity- avoid slopes as you won't be doing much.

Swimming

Swimming is a full-body cardio workout. The burn begins when you get into the water, as you are essentially fighting gravity with your muscles to keep afloat. Just a minute of swimming burns you 14 calories; just be sure to incorporate different strokes as each stroke has a different level of intensity.

Other fun activity cardio you can try out include:

- *Dancing*
- *Boxing*
- *Power walking*
- *Organized sports*
- *Trampoline-ing*
- *Hiking*
- *Rowing*
- *Hula-hooping*
- *Walking*
- *Jumping jacks*

2: Strength Training

This is any form of exercise that uses resistance to induce muscular contractions. These contractions, in turn, burn fat, build muscle and strength. Strength training can be explained further by these 2 actions:

The movement of weight- As long as you are utilizing weights (or even your body weight) to work out, then this is strength training.

Progressive overload- If you increase your efforts compared to your previous workout consistently, then this is also strength training (e.g., using heavier weights or increasing workout reps).

Strength Training Exercises

Lunges

A lunge involves standing upright and moving one leg forward as you bend your knee. There are many variations to a lunge, such as a backward lunge (moving your leg backward) or a curtsy lunge (a sideways lunge).

Lunges tone your legs and glutes and are great for improving balance.

Squats

Squats are famously known for building 'the booty', but they are also a great leg work out. To perform a squat, stand upright with your feet shoulder-width apart. Squat as if sitting on an imaginary chair and then push back up.

There are also different variations of squats such as a jump squat (where you do a squat, then jump back up), sumo squat (where you squat with your legs wide open), squat and kick (you squat and kick one leg sideways), etc.

Push-ups

Push-ups are a popular exercise for toning arms and building arm strength. To perform a push-up, move to a plank position, lower your elbows as far as you can, keep your back straight, and then push back up.

There are also different variations of a push up such as knee push-ups and wall push-ups (try these if you are a beginner), shoulder taps (where you perform a push-up and then tap your shoulders in plank position), single-leg push up (a push up with one leg raised), etc.

Exercising with dumbbells or kettlebells

You can literally make any type of exercise strength training by incorporating weights. If you want to build intensity, pick up weights, and perform your workouts with them.

Now that you understand the workouts you should perform to increase your body's energy requirements and have already understood dieting for weight loss, what you need now is the motivation to keep going, even when the results don't seem to come overnight.

Chapter 4: How To Stay Motivated

Sometimes we really want to do something but lack the willpower or time to do it - trust me, you are not alone. When it comes to exercising, the more you work out, the more you will love working out. The beginning is always the hardest (sore muscles, anyone?).

As you continue working out, you will notice your efforts bearing fruit, you will have more energy and you won't struggle too much with the exercises - so just hold on a little longer.

The same applies to changing your diet - as you stick to your new diet, you will notice how great you feel and look.

But just how do you get there?

Do it for you - Find internal motivation. Why do you want to lose weight? How will you feel after achieving your dream weight? How happy will you be? Picture yourself at your dream weight. How will you feel? Remember that in the end, you are doing this for yourself and that you are working hard to live a healthier life.

Go slow - If you start with a really intense and hard work out, it will be easy for you to give up. If you eliminate all the unhealthy foods at once, it will be hard on you, and it will be so easy for you to relapse. Make sure you take things slow. For your diet, you can try and eliminate one food at a time until you get rid of all the unhealthy foods from your diet. For your workouts, follow the guidelines, as indicated in the book.

Do what suits you best - Whether it's a diet or a workout regime, go with one that works for you. If you prefer working out in the evening, do that; if you prefer fasting for a whole day but twice a week compared to every day then do that. The point is to make your weight loss journey as comfortable as you can so that it can feel more like part of your lifestyle.

The more, the merrier - A workout/dieting partner can help you get back in the right direction. Find someone that has the same goals as you and take them on your journey. Set goals together and work hard to achieve them together. It is so easy to stay motivated when you have someone by your side.

Go easy on yourself- Remember that you can never be perfect. Missed a few workouts? It's okay. Had an extra cookie? It's okay too. Don't beat yourself up if you go astray every once in a while because it will happen, and it does happen. And when it does happen, acknowledge it did and then go back to your awesome healthy living.

Conclusion

The best way to lose weight and keep it off is by combining dieting and exercising. But make sure to start slow so that you don't give up, even before you start. Go easy on yourself and enjoy the journey!

www.ingramcontent.com/pod-product-compliance
Lightning Source LLC
Chambersburg PA
CBHW061547250726
48657CB00006B/2334